I0705064

Smoothie Solutions:

Thyroid Healing with Delicious Blends.

By Donna Nettles

All rights reserved. No part of this book may be reproduced in any form or by any electronic or mechanical means, including information storage and retrieval systems, without permission in writing from the publisher, except by a reviewer who may quote brief passages in a review.

Copyright © 2023 by Donna Nettles

TABLE OF CONTENTS

INTRODUCTION

Tom had been struggling with his thyroid for years and was feeling like he was out of options. He had tried countless treatments, medications, and even some alternative therapies, but nothing seemed to fully help him. He was feeling frustrated and exhausted with his condition, and was beginning to lose hope.

That's when he stumbled across a blog post about thyroid healing with smoothies. He was intrigued but wasn't sure if it was something he should try. After doing some research, he decided to give it a chance.

Tom began by changing his diet and adding more fresh fruits and vegetables to his meals. He also started drinking smoothies made with ingredients known to help support thyroid health, like spinach, kale, coconut oil, and almond milk. In addition, he began taking supplements to support his thyroid and help bring his hormones back into balance.

Within just a few weeks, Tom began to notice a difference in his energy levels and general well-being. The smoothies seemed to be helping him feel better and his hormones were gradually coming back into balance.

After a few months, Tom was feeling better than he had in years. His energy levels were back to normal, he wasn't experiencing any of the symptoms of hypothyroidism, and his overall health had improved.

Tom was amazed by the transformation and couldn't believe how much of a difference the smoothies had made. He was so pleased with his results that he started sharing his story with others, in the hope that it might help them too.

Tom's success story is an inspiration to anyone struggling with thyroid health. It shows that, with the right diet and lifestyle changes, it is possible to heal your thyroid and improve your quality of life.

THYROID HEALING

Thyroid healing involves treating the underlying cause of thyroid dysfunction, such as an autoimmune condition, and restoring the body's balance of hormones. This is usually done through dietary changes, lifestyle modifications, and natural supplements. Additionally, practitioners may employ other therapies such as acupuncture, meditation, and homeopathy to help with healing and restoration.

Healing the thyroid naturally is possible and can be a beneficial, non-invasive way to restore balance to your body. The thyroid is an important gland in the body that helps regulate metabolism and other bodily functions, so restoring balance to it is essential for overall health.

One of the most important steps to healing the thyroid naturally is to ensure that you are getting adequate nutrition and hydration. Eating a balanced diet of fresh, whole foods and avoiding processed foods can help supply your body with the vitamins and minerals it needs to function optimally. Additionally, drinking plenty of water and avoiding sugar and caffeine can help keep your body hydrated and reduce inflammation.

Supplementation can also be beneficial in healing the thyroid naturally. Certain vitamins and minerals, such as iodine, selenium, zinc, and vitamin B12, are important for healthy thyroid function. Additionally, herbs such as ashwagandha, turmeric, and holy basil can help regulate thyroid hormones and reduce inflammation.

Finally, stress management and getting adequate sleep are essential for thyroid health as well.

Stress can disrupt hormone balance, so finding effective ways to manage it, such as through yoga, meditation, or deep breathing exercises, can help support thyroid health.

Smoothies are a delicious and nutritious way to support thyroid health. Smoothies are an easy way to get the essential nutrients necessary for thyroid healing, including vitamins, minerals, and antioxidants. The natural ingredients in smoothies can help to reduce inflammation, boost your energy, and aid in hormone regulation. Smoothies are also a great way to get essential omega-3 fatty acids, which are important for thyroid function. Additionally, smoothies can provide prebiotics and probiotics which can help to restore the balance of gut bacteria, which is crucial for thyroid health.

The nutrients found in smoothies can help to reduce the risk of thyroid disease, as well as provide relief for those who already have a thyroid disorder. Smoothies are an easy way to get all of the essential vitamins, minerals, and antioxidants needed for thyroid health. Smoothies can also provide omega-3 fatty acids, which are important for maintaining proper thyroid function. Additionally, smoothies can provide prebiotics and probiotics which can help to restore the balance of gut bacteria, which is crucial for thyroid health.

When creating a smoothie for thyroid healing, it is important to include nutrient-dense ingredients such as leafy greens, avocados, nuts, seeds, and nut butter. It's also important to include ingredients that contain iodine, such as seafood, seaweed, and iodized salt. Additionally, adding superfoods that are high in antioxidants such as blueberries, goji berries, and acai can help to reduce inflammation and protect against oxidative stress.

To make a delicious and nutritious smoothie for thyroid healing, blend leafy greens, avocado, nuts, seeds, nut butter, and frozen fruit. Add a few slices of fresh ginger for a spicy kick, and a few tablespoons of coconut oil for added healthy fats. For extra flavor and nutrition, add superfoods such as blueberries, goji berries, and acai. Finally, top off your smoothie with a handful of ice and some filtered water or unsweetened almond milk.

By making a nutrient-dense smoothie for thyroid healing, you can get the essential vitamins, minerals, and antioxidants needed for optimal thyroid health. Smoothies are an easy and delicious way to support your thyroid and keep it functioning optimally.

CHAPTER 1: Understanding The Thyroid

The thyroid is a small, butterfly-shaped gland located at the front of the neck, just below the Adam's apple. It is an essential part of the endocrine system and is responsible for producing hormones that regulate metabolism and energy levels. The hormones produced by the thyroid are called triiodothyronine (T3) and thyroxine (T4).

The thyroid gland is part of the endocrine system, which is responsible for producing hormones that regulate many different body functions. T4 and T3 are produced from the amino acid tyrosine and are regulated by the pituitary gland in the brain. The pituitary gland releases the hormones TSH (thyroid stimulating hormone) and TRH (thyrotropin-releasing hormone), which signal the thyroid to produce and release T4 and T3.

The main function of the thyroid is to regulate the body's metabolism. Metabolism is the process by which the body transforms food into energy. When thyroid hormones are produced and released, they travel through the bloodstream and act on the cells in the body.

When the thyroid is not producing sufficient hormones, this is known as hypothyroidism. Symptoms of hypothyroidism can include fatigue, weight gain, depression, dry skin, and constipation. On the other hand, when the thyroid produces too much hormone, this is known as hyperthyroidism. Symptoms of hyperthyroidism can include anxiety, weight loss, irritability, tremors, and irregular heartbeat.

CAUSES OF THYROID DISEASES/PROBLEMS

To diagnose and treat thyroid conditions, it is important to understand how the thyroid works and what can cause it to malfunction. The thyroid is regulated by a hormone called thyroid-stimulating hormone (TSH), which is produced by the pituitary gland in the brain. When TSH levels are too low, the thyroid does not produce enough hormones, resulting in hypothyroidism. When TSH levels are too high, the thyroid produces too much hormone, resulting in hyperthyroidism.

Thyroid conditions can be caused by a variety of factors, including autoimmune disorders, medications, radiation therapy, infections, nutritional deficiencies, stress, age, environmental factors, and genetic disorders.
Other thyroid disorders include hyperthyroidism, goiter, and thyroid cancer.

Genetics

Genetic factors are a common cause of thyroid problems, particularly autoimmune thyroid disorders. In autoimmune thyroid disorders, the immune system attacks the thyroid gland, leading to either hypothyroidism or hyperthyroidism. These conditions can be caused by inherited genetic mutations that disrupt the functioning of the immune system. Some genetic mutations can also directly affect the thyroid gland, leading to problems with hormone production.

Autoimmune Conditions

Autoimmune conditions are a common cause of thyroid problems, particularly Hashimoto's thyroiditis and Graves' disease. In Hashimoto's thyroiditis, the immune system attacks the thyroid gland, resulting in it not producing enough hormones, leading to hypothyroidism. Graves' disease is an autoimmune condition in which the immune system stimulates the thyroid gland to produce too much hormone, leading to hyperthyroidism.

Environmental Factors

Certain environmental factors can also lead to thyroid problems. For example, exposure to certain chemicals, such as polychlorinated biphenyls (PCBs), can disrupt the functioning of the thyroid gland, leading to hypothyroidism. Radiation exposure, such as that from radiation therapy for cancer, can also damage the thyroid gland and lead to both hyperthyroidism and hypothyroidism.

Infections

Infections can also lead to thyroid problems. For example, certain viruses, such as the Epstein-Barr virus, can cause the thyroid gland to become inflamed, leading to hypothyroidism. Bacterial infections, such as those caused by Streptococcus, can also cause inflammation of the thyroid gland.

Medications

Certain medications, such as lithium and interferon-alpha, can also cause thyroid problems. These medications can interfere with the production of thyroid hormones, leading to either hypothyroidism or hyperthyroidism.

Nutritional Deficiencies

Nutritional deficiencies can also cause thyroid problems. For example, a lack of iodine can lead to hypothyroidism, as the body needs iodine to produce thyroid hormones. A lack of selenium can also lead to thyroid problems, as selenium is necessary for the production of thyroid hormones.

Stress

Stress can also lead to thyroid problems. Stress can disrupt the body's hormones and interfere with the functioning of the thyroid gland, leading to either hypothyroidism or hyperthyroidism.

Age

Age can also lead to thyroid problems. As people age, the thyroid gland can become less efficient at producing thyroid hormones, leading to hypothyroidism. Thyroid cancer is also more common in older adults.

To diagnose and treat a thyroid disorder, your doctor may order blood tests to measure TSH, T3, and T4 levels. If the results indicate that your thyroid is not functioning properly, your doctor may prescribe medication to adjust the levels of hormones in your body. Additional treatments may include radiation therapy, surgery, and lifestyle changes.

It is important to understand the role of the thyroid to maintain optimal health. If you are experiencing any of the symptoms mentioned above, it is important to speak to your doctor about potential thyroid disorders. With the proper diagnosis and treatment, most thyroid conditions can be managed.

CHAPTER 2: Benefits Of Smoothies For Thyroid Health

Smoothies are a great way to get a variety of essential nutrients into your body, and they offer many benefits for thyroid health. Fortunately, smoothies can help to promote healthy thyroid function. The main ingredients in smoothies—fruits and vegetables—are rich in antioxidants, vitamins, and minerals that are essential for maintaining a healthy thyroid. Antioxidants protect the cells from damage caused by free radicals and help to reduce inflammation. Vitamins and minerals like selenium, zinc, and iodine support the thyroid's ability to produce hormones.

Smoothies can also provide your body with healthy fats, like omega-3s. These fats help to reduce inflammation, which is often linked to thyroid disorders. Additionally, healthy fats can help to improve your mood, which can be beneficial if you're dealing with depression or anxiety.

Smoothies are also a great way to get more fiber into your diet. Fiber helps your body to process and eliminate toxins, which can help to reduce the risk of thyroid disorders. Fiber also helps to keep your blood sugar levels stable, which is important for maintaining healthy thyroid function.

Smoothies are also a great way to get more protein into your diet. Protein helps to boost your metabolic rate and helps your body to absorb other nutrients more effectively. Protein is also important for maintaining healthy muscles, which can help to reduce fatigue.

Finally, smoothies are a great way to get more vitamins and minerals into your diet. Vitamins and minerals like vitamin D, iron, magnesium, and calcium are all important for maintaining healthy thyroid function. Smoothies are a great way to get these essential nutrients without having to take supplements.

In Summary,

1. Smoothies are packed with fiber, which can help regulate thyroid hormones.
2. They can contain healthy fats like avocado, chia seeds, flaxseed, and coconut, which help to support hormone production and balance.
3. They are a great source of iodine, a mineral that is essential for healthy thyroid function.
4. Smoothies are a good source of B vitamins, which help to support overall thyroid health.
5. They are full of antioxidants, which can help to protect the thyroid gland from damage.
6. They can contain adaptogens and herbs that help to regulate hormone production and balance.
7. Smoothies contain essential minerals like magnesium, zinc, and selenium, which can help the thyroid to function optimally.

8. They are a great way to get plenty of fruits and vegetables, which can provide the body with key vitamins and minerals for thyroid health.
9. Smoothies are a delicious and convenient way to get the nutrients your body needs to support thyroid health.
10. They provide a great source of energy, which can help to reduce fatigue and improve thyroid health.

Overall, smoothies offer many health benefits for thyroid health. Not only do they provide essential nutrients, but they are also quick and easy to make. So next time you're looking to give your thyroid a boost, try making a smoothie!

CHAPTER 3: The Best Ingredients For Thyroid Health

When it comes to thyroid health, the right ingredients can make all the difference. Fortunately, there are a variety of natural ingredients that can help to restore and maintain thyroid health. These ingredients are rich in essential nutrients, such as iodine, zinc, selenium, and vitamins A, E, and C. They can also help to boost energy levels, balance hormones, and even reduce inflammation. Here are some of the best ingredients for thyroid health.

Iodine: Iodine is a key ingredient for thyroid health, as it helps to produce hormones that regulate metabolism. It can be found in sea vegetables, such as seaweed and kelp, as well as in iodized salt.

Zinc: Zinc is an essential mineral for thyroid health and can help to regulate the production of hormones. It can be found in foods such as oysters, beef, peanuts, and pumpkin seeds.

Selenium: Selenium is a mineral that helps to activate enzymes in the thyroid and is important for the production of hormones. It can be found in Brazil nuts, mushrooms, tuna, and eggs.

Vitamins A, E, and C: These vitamins are essential for the proper functioning of the thyroid, as they help to regulate hormone levels. Vitamin A can be found in carrots, sweet potatoes, and spinach, while Vitamin E is found in nuts and seeds, and Vitamin C is found in citrus fruits, tomatoes, and bell peppers.

Turmeric: Turmeric is a popular spice that has anti-inflammatory properties and can help to reduce inflammation in the thyroid. It can be found in curry powders and is also available in supplement form.

Garlic: Garlic contains sulfur-containing compounds that can help the body to produce hormones, making it a great ingredient for thyroid health. It can be added to a variety of dishes or taken in supplement form.

Ginger: Ginger is another spice that has anti-inflammatory properties and can help to reduce inflammation in the thyroid. It can be added to smoothies, teas, and dishes or taken in supplement form.

Ashwagandha: This herb helps to reduce stress levels and balance hormones.

Probiotics: Probiotics are beneficial bacteria that help to restore balance to the gut microbiome.

Cruciferous Vegetables: These vegetables, such as broccoli and kale, contain compounds that help to detoxify the body.

Selenium-Rich Foods: Selenium is a mineral that helps to activate enzymes in the thyroid, and foods such as brazil nuts, oysters, and tuna are rich in it.

Brazil Nuts: These nuts are a great source of selenium and can help to regulate the production of hormones.

Almonds: Almonds are a great source of zinc and can help to balance hormones.

Maca: This root vegetable contains minerals that help to support the adrenal glands and balance hormones.

MCT Oil: This oil contains medium-chain triglycerides that can help to boost energy levels.

Coconut Oil: Coconut oil is a huge source of healthy fats and can help to regulate hormones.

Green Tea: Green tea is packed with antioxidants and can help to boost energy levels.

Omega-3 Fatty Acids: These fatty acids can help to reduce inflammation and balance hormones.

Probiotic-Rich Foods: Foods such as yogurt, kefir, sauerkraut, and kimchi contain beneficial bacteria that can help to restore balance to the gut microbiome.

Probiotic Supplements: These supplements provide beneficial bacteria to help restore balance to the gut microbiome.

Spirulina: This blue-green alga is packed with nutrients and can help to reduce inflammation.

Goji Berries: These berries are rich in antioxidants and can help to reduce inflammation.

Incorporating these ingredients into your diet can help to restore and maintain thyroid health and prevent a variety of issues. In addition, it's important to consult with your healthcare provider to determine the best approach for your needs.

CHAPTER 4: Tips For Preparing Delicious And Nutritious Smoothies For Thyroid Health

When it comes to preparing delicious and nutritious smoothies for thyroid health, there are some key tips that you should keep in mind. Smoothies are a great way to get the vitamins and minerals you need to maintain your thyroid health, as well as the energy to get through the day. Here are some tips for preparing delicious and nutritious smoothies for thyroid health.

1. Include Healthy Fats

Healthy fats are essential for proper thyroid function and overall health. When preparing your smoothie, be sure to include healthy fats such as coconut oil, avocado, nuts, or nut butter. These healthy fats will help to regulate your hormones and improve your overall health.

2. Add Protein

Protein is also essential for maintaining good thyroid health. You can add protein to your smoothie by adding Greek yogurt, milk, or protein powder. Doing so will help to keep you full and satisfied for hours, as well as provide the building blocks for your cells and hormones.

3. Include Leafy Greens

Leafy greens are an important part of any diet, but especially so for those with thyroid issues. Leafy greens are packed with vitamins and minerals that are essential for proper thyroid function. Spinach and kale are two of the best options, but you can also add romaine, arugula, and Swiss chard.

4. Get Creative with Your Ingredients

Smoothies are the perfect way to get creative with your ingredients and make them as delicious and nutritious as possible. You can add fruits, vegetables, nuts, seeds, spices, and even superfoods. Some great superfoods to add to your smoothies include maca, chia seeds, and Acai powder.

5. Use Healthy Sweeteners

When preparing your smoothie, it's important to use healthy sweeteners. Refined sugar can be detrimental to your thyroid health, so try to avoid it when possible. Instead, opt for natural or raw sweeteners such as honey, maple syrup, or dates.

6. Include Healthy Herbs

Including healthy herbs in your smoothie can help to improve your thyroid health. Adaptogenic herbs such as ashwagandha, reishi, and maca are especially beneficial. These herbs help to balance your hormones, reduce stress, and boost energy.

7. Start with a Base

When preparing your smoothie, it is best to start with a base such as almond milk, coconut milk, or oat milk. This will help to make your smoothie creamy and delicious. You can also add a banana, avocado, Greek yogurt, or nut butter to make your smoothie even creamier.

8. Take Your Time

When preparing your smoothie, it is important to take your time and be mindful of the process. This will help to ensure that your smoothie is full of flavor and nutrition. Take your time to pick out the best ingredients and experiment with different combinations.

When it comes to preparing delicious and nutritious smoothies for thyroid health, it's important to keep these tips in mind. By following these tips, you can ensure that your smoothies are full of flavor and nutrition, and provide the vitamins and minerals you need for proper thyroid health.

CHAPTER 5: 30 Delicious And Nutritious Smoothie Recipes For Thyroid Health

1. Apple Pie Smoothie:

Ingredients:

2 cups unsweetened almond milk

2 scoops vanilla protein powder

1 apple, cored and diced

1/2 teaspoon ground cinnamon

1/2 teaspoon ground nutmeg

1/4 teaspoon ground ginger

1/4 teaspoon ground allspice

1 tablespoon of honey

Method: Place all ingredients in a blender and blend until desired consistency is reached.

Storage: Store any leftovers in an airtight bottle in the refrigerator for up to 3 days.

2. Strawberry-Banana Smoothie:

<u>Ingredients:</u>

1 cup unsweetened almond milk

1 scoop vanilla protein powder

1 cup fresh strawberries

1 banana

1/2 teaspoon ground cinnamon

1 tablespoon honey

<u>Method:</u> Place all ingredients in a blender and blend until desired consistency is reached.

<u>Storage:</u> Store any leftovers in an airtight bottle in the refrigerator for up to 3 days.

3. Mango-Pineapple Smoothie:

<u>Ingredients:</u>

2 cups unsweetened almond milk

2 scoops vanilla protein powder

1 cup diced mango

1/2 cup diced pineapple

1/2 teaspoon ground turmeric

1 tablespoon honey

Method: Place all ingredients in a blender and blend until desired consistency is reached.

Storage: Store any leftovers in an airtight bottle in the refrigerator for up to 3 days.

4. Green Tea-Kale Smoothie:

Ingredients: 1 cup of unsweetened almond milk

 1 scoop vanilla protein powder

1 cup kale

 1/2 teaspoon matcha green tea powder

1/2 teaspoon ground turmeric

 1 tablespoon honey

Method: Place all ingredients in a blender and blend until desired consistency is reached.

Storage: Store any leftovers in an airtight bottle in the refrigerator for up to 3 days.

5. Blueberry-Oat Smoothie:

Ingredients:

2 cups unsweetened almond milk

1 scoop vanilla protein powder

 1/2 cup old-fashioned oats

1 cup fresh or frozen blueberries

1/2 teaspoon ground cinnamon
1 tablespoon honey

<u>Method:</u> Place all ingredients in a blender and blend until desired consistency is reached.
<u>Storage:</u> Store any leftovers in an airtight bottle in the refrigerator for up to 3 days.

6. Avocado-Papaya Smoothie:

<u>Ingredients:</u>
1 cup unsweetened almond milk
1 scoop vanilla protein powder
1/2 avocado, peeled and pitted
1 cup diced papaya
1/2 teaspoon ground ginger
1 tablespoon honey

<u>Method:</u> Place all ingredients in a blender and blend until desired consistency is reached.
<u>Storage:</u> Store any leftovers in an airtight bottle in the refrigerator for up to 3 days.

7. Chocolate-Mint Smoothie:

Ingredients:
 2 cups unsweetened almond milk
 2 scoops vanilla protein powder
 2 tablespoons unsweetened cocoa powder
1/2 teaspoon peppermint extract
 1 tablespoon honey

Method: Place all ingredients in a blender and blend until desired consistency is reached.
Storage: Store any leftovers in an airtight bottle in the refrigerator for up to 3 days.

8. Cherry-Almond Smoothie:

Ingredients:
1 cup unsweetened almond milk
 1 scoop vanilla protein powder
 1 cup pitted cherries
 1/4 cup almonds
 1/2 teaspoon ground cinnamon
1 tablespoon honey

Method: Place all ingredients in a blender and blend until desired consistency is reached.

<u>Storage:</u> Store any leftovers in an airtight bottle in the refrigerator for up to 3 days.

9. Peach-Coconut Smoothie:

<u>Ingredients:</u>

2 cups unsweetened almond milk

2 scoops vanilla protein powder

1 cup diced peaches

1/4 cup shredded coconut

1/2 teaspoon ground ginger

1 tablespoon honey

<u>Method:</u> Place all ingredients in a blender and blend until desired consistency is reached.

<u>Storage:</u> Store any leftovers in an airtight bottle in the refrigerator for up to 3 days.

10. Pear-Ginger Smoothie:

<u>Ingredients:</u>

1 cup unsweetened almond milk

1 scoop vanilla protein powder

1 pear, cored and diced

1/2 teaspoon ground ginger

1 tablespoon honey

Method: Place all ingredients in a blender and blend until desired consistency is reached.
Storage: Store any leftovers in an airtight bottle in the refrigerator for up to 3 days.

11. Coconut-Lemon Smoothie:

Ingredients:
2 cups unsweetened almond milk
 2 scoops vanilla protein powder
 1/4 cup shredded coconut
 1/2 teaspoon ground turmeric
 1 tablespoon honey
juice of 1 lemon

Method: Place all ingredients in a blender and blend until desired consistency is reached.
Storage: Store any leftovers in an airtight bottle in the refrigerator for up to 3 days.

12. Banana-Almond Butter Smoothie:

Ingredients:
1 cup unsweetened almond milk
1 scoop vanilla protein powder
1 banana

2 tablespoons almond butter
1/2 teaspoon ground cinnamon
1 tablespoon honey

<u>Method:</u> Place all ingredients in a blender and blend until desired consistency is reached.
<u>Storage:</u> Store any leftovers in an airtight bottle in the refrigerator for up to 3 days.

13. Carrot-Orange Smoothie:
<u>Ingredients:</u>
2 cups unsweetened almond milk
 2 scoops vanilla protein powder
 1 cup grated carrots
1/2 cup fresh orange juice
1/2 teaspoon ground turmeric
1 tablespoon honey

<u>Method:</u> Place all ingredients in a blender and blend until desired consistency is reached.
<u>Storage:</u> Store any leftovers in an airtight bottle in the refrigerator for up to 3 days.

14. Grape-Vanilla Smoothie:

<u>Ingredients:</u>

1 cup unsweetened almond milk

1 scoop vanilla protein powder

1 cup red grapes

2 teaspoons pure vanilla extract

1/2 teaspoon ground cinnamon

1 tablespoon honey

<u>Method:</u> Place all ingredients in a blender and blend until desired consistency is reached.

<u>Storage:</u> Store any leftovers in an airtight bottle in the refrigerator for up to 3 days.

15. Apricot-Ginger Smoothie:

<u>Ingredients:</u>

2 cups unsweetened almond milk

2 scoops vanilla protein powder

1 cup diced apricots

1/2 teaspoon ground ginger

1 tablespoon honey

<u>Method:</u> Place all ingredients in a blender and blend until desired consistency is reached.

Storage: Store any leftovers in an airtight bottle in the refrigerator for up to 3 days.

16. Kiwi-Mint Smoothie:

Ingredients:

1 cup unsweetened almond milk

1 scoop vanilla protein powder

1 kiwi peeled and diced

1/2 teaspoon peppermint extract

1 tablespoon honey

Method: Place all ingredients in a blender and blend until desired consistency is reached.

Storage: Store any leftovers in an airtight bottle in the refrigerator for up to 3 days.

17. Pumpkin-Spice Smoothie:

Ingredients:

2 cups unsweetened almond milk

2 scoops vanilla protein powder

1/2 cup canned pumpkin puree

1/2 teaspoon ground cinnamon

1/4 teaspoon ground nutmeg

1/4 teaspoon ground ginger

1/4 teaspoon ground allspice

1 tablespoon honey

Method: Place all ingredients in a blender and blend until desired consistency is reached.

Storage: Store any leftovers in an airtight bottle in the refrigerator for up to 3 days.

18. Banana-Spinach Smoothie:

Ingredients:

1 cup unsweetened almond milk

1 scoop vanilla protein powder

1 banana

1 cup fresh spinach

1/2 teaspoon ground turmeric

1 tablespoon honey

Method: Place all ingredients in a blender and blend until desired consistency is reached.

Storage: Store any leftovers in an airtight bottle in the refrigerator for up to 3 days.

19. Mango-Coconut Smoothie:

<u>Ingredients:</u>

2 cups unsweetened almond milk

2 scoops vanilla protein powder

1 cup diced mango

1/4 cup shredded coconut

1/2 teaspoon ground ginger

1 tablespoon honey

<u>Method:</u> Place all ingredients in a blender and blend until desired consistency is reached.

<u>Storage:</u> Store any leftovers in an airtight bottle in the refrigerator for up to 3 days.

20. Apple-Cinnamon Smoothie:

<u>Ingredients:</u>

1 cup unsweetened almond milk

1 scoop vanilla protein powder

1 apple, cored and diced

1/2 teaspoon ground cinnamon

1 tablespoon honey

<u>Method:</u> Place all ingredients in a blender and blend until desired consistency is reached.

Storage: Store any leftovers in an airtight bottle in the refrigerator for up to 3 days.

21. Watermelon-Lime Smoothie:
Ingredients:
2 cups unsweetened almond milk
 2 scoops vanilla protein powder
1 cup diced watermelon
juice of 1 lime
1/2 teaspoon ground turmeric
1 tablespoon honey

Method: Place all ingredients in a blender and blend until desired consistency is reached.
Storage: Store any leftovers in an airtight bottle in the refrigerator for up to 3 days.

22. Orange-Ginger Smoothie:
Ingredients:
1 cup unsweetened almond milk
1 scoop vanilla protein powder
1/2 cup fresh orange juice
 1/2 teaspoon ground ginger
1 tablespoon honey

<u>Method:</u> Place all ingredients in a blender and blend until desired consistency is reached.

<u>Storage:</u> Store any leftovers in an airtight bottle in the refrigerator for up to 3 days.

23. Raspberry-Vanilla Smoothie:

<u>Ingredients:</u>

2 cups unsweetened almond milk

2 scoops vanilla protein powder

1 cup fresh or frozen raspberries

2 teaspoons pure vanilla extract

1/2 teaspoon ground cinnamon

1 tablespoon honey

<u>Method:</u> Place all ingredients in a blender and blend until desired consistency is reached.

<u>Storage:</u> Store any leftovers in an airtight bottle in the refrigerator for up to 3 days.

24. Pineapple-Mango Smoothie:

<u>Ingredients:</u>

1 cup unsweetened almond milk

1 scoop vanilla protein powder

1/2 cup diced pineapple

1/2 cup diced mango
1/2 teaspoon ground turmeric
1 tablespoon honey

<u>Method:</u> Place all ingredients in a blender and blend until desired consistency is reached.
<u>Storage:</u> Store any leftovers in an airtight bottle in the refrigerator for up to 3 days.

25. Peach-Pecan Smoothie:
<u>Ingredients:</u>
2 cups unsweetened almond milk
 2 scoops vanilla protein powder
 1 cup diced peaches
 1/4 cup pecans
 1/2 teaspoon ground cinnamon
1 tablespoon honey

<u>Method:</u> Place all ingredients in a blender and blend until desired consistency is reached.
<u>Storage:</u> Store any leftovers in an airtight bottle in the refrigerator for up to 3 days.

26. Apricot-Coconut Smoothie:

<u>Ingredients:</u>

1 cup unsweetened almond milk

1 scoop vanilla protein powder

1 cup diced apricots

1/4 cup shredded coconut

1/2 teaspoon ground ginger

1 tablespoon honey

<u>Method:</u> Place all ingredients in a blender and blend until desired consistency is reached.

<u>Storage:</u> Store any leftovers in an airtight bottle in the refrigerator for up to 3 days.

27. Apple-Cranberry Smoothie:

<u>Ingredients:</u>

2 cups unsweetened almond milk

2 scoops vanilla protein powder

1 apple, cored and diced

1/2 cup fresh or frozen cranberries

1/2 teaspoon ground cinnamon

1 tablespoon honey

<u>Method:</u> Place all ingredients in a blender and blend until desired consistency is reached.

<u>Storage:</u> Store any leftovers in an airtight bottle in the refrigerator for up to 3 days.

28. Carrot-Cherry Smoothie:

<u>Ingredients:</u>

1 cup unsweetened almond milk

1 scoop vanilla protein powder

1 cup grated carrots

1/2 cup pitted cherries

1/2 teaspoon ground turmeric

1 tablespoon honey

<u>Method:</u> Place all ingredients in a blender and blend until desired consistency is reached.

<u>Storage:</u> Store any leftovers in an airtight bottle in the refrigerator for up to 3 days.

29. Grapefruit-Mint Smoothie:

<u>Ingredients:</u>

2 cups unsweetened almond milk

2 scoops vanilla protein powder

1/2 cup fresh grapefruit juice

1/2 teaspoon peppermint extract
1 tablespoon honey

Method: Place all ingredients in a blender and blend until desired consistency is reached.
Storage: Store any leftovers in an airtight bottle in the refrigerator for up to 3 days.

30. Banana-Almond Smoothie:
Ingredients:
1 cup unsweetened almond milk
1 scoop vanilla protein powder
1 banana
1/4 cup almonds
1/2 teaspoon ground cinnamon
1 tablespoon honey

Method: Place all ingredients in a blender and blend until desired consistency is reached.
Storage: Store any leftovers in an airtight bottle in the refrigerator for up to 3 days.

CHAPTER 6: Tips For Staying On Track With Smoothies

Smoothies are a great way to get all the nutrients you need to stay healthy and keep your thyroid functioning properly. Your thyroid plays an important role in regulating your metabolism, energy levels, and overall health. When it isn't functioning properly, you may experience fatigue, weight gain, and other health issues. By following these tips for staying on track with smoothies for thyroid health, you can help ensure that your thyroid is functioning properly and that you're getting the right nutrients to stay healthy and energized.

1. Use organic ingredients whenever possible.
Organic ingredients are not only better for the environment but they're also better for you. Organic produce is free from pesticides, synthetic fertilizers, and other contaminants that can interfere with your thyroid health and hormone levels. Choose organic ingredients

whenever possible for your smoothies and you'll
be doing your body a favor.

2. Include healthy fats.
Healthy fats are important for thyroid health and
can help the body absorb essential nutrients like
iodine. Try adding a few tablespoons of coconut
oil, flaxseed oil, or avocado oil to your
smoothies. You can also add nuts like almonds
or walnuts, nut butter, and seeds like chia or
hemp for an extra boost of healthy fats.

3. Include iodine-rich foods.
Iodine is an important mineral for thyroid health
and can be found in foods like seaweed, fish,
eggs, and dairy products. You can easily add
these ingredients to your smoothies to help
support your thyroid health. Try adding a few
pieces of seaweed, a tablespoon of fish oil, or a
few tablespoons of yogurt to your smoothies.

4. Add leafy greens.
Leafy greens are packed with vitamins, minerals,
and antioxidants that can help keep your thyroid

functioning properly. Try adding kale, spinach, collard greens, or Swiss chard to your smoothies for an extra boost of nutrition.

5. Include vitamin B.

Vitamin B is important for thyroid health and can be found in foods like eggs, meat, fish, and dairy products. You can also get your daily dose of vitamin B from fortified foods like breakfast cereals. Add a few tablespoons of these ingredients to your smoothies to get the vitamin B you need for healthy thyroid functioning.

6. Include herbs and spices.

Herbs and spices are loaded with antioxidants and other nutrients that can help support your thyroid health. Try adding a teaspoon of cinnamon, turmeric, ginger, or cumin to your smoothies for an extra boost of flavor and nutrition.

7. Drink plenty of water.

Staying hydrated is important for your overall health, including your thyroid health. Make sure you're drinking plenty of water throughout the day to help keep your thyroid functioning properly.

By following these tips for staying on track with smoothies for thyroid health, you can help ensure that your thyroid is functioning properly and that you're getting the right nutrients to stay healthy and energized. Whether you're trying to lose weight, gain energy, or just stay healthy, smoothies can be a great way to get the nutrients you need. With the right ingredients, you can create delicious, nutritious smoothies that will help you stay on track and keep your thyroid functioning properly.

CONCLUSION

The journey of learning about the power of smoothies for thyroid health has been an enlightening one. From understanding how to leverage the many vitamins, minerals, and antioxidants found in fruits and vegetables, to the invaluable benefits of adding superfoods, herbs, and spices, smoothies provide an easy and delicious way to support and improve thyroid health. Not only do smoothies taste great and can be tailored to fit any dietary preference or lifestyle, but they can also be beneficial for those with thyroid issues, helping to reduce inflammation, regulate hormones, and improve energy levels.

Smoothies can be an excellent part of a healthy diet for anyone, but for those with thyroid issues, they can be an especially valuable resource. By utilizing the advice and recipes found in this book, you can start to enjoy the many benefits of thyroid-friendly smoothies. Whether you're looking to prevent or manage a thyroid disorder, or just want to enjoy some delicious, health-boosting smoothies, the knowledge, and recipes in this book will help you get started. With a bit of experimentation and customization, you can find the right smoothies for you, so that you can achieve and maintain optimal thyroid health.

Also, don't forget that dietary changes should always be discussed with your doctor and you should always consult a healthcare professional to ensure that your diet and lifestyle are supporting your individual needs. By becoming aware of and mindful of the food choices available to you, you can make the most of your health and well-being.

By following the advice and recipes in this book, you can start to reap the many benefits that smoothies can provide for thyroid health. With delicious, nutrient-packed smoothies, you can support your thyroid health and enjoy a healthier lifestyle.

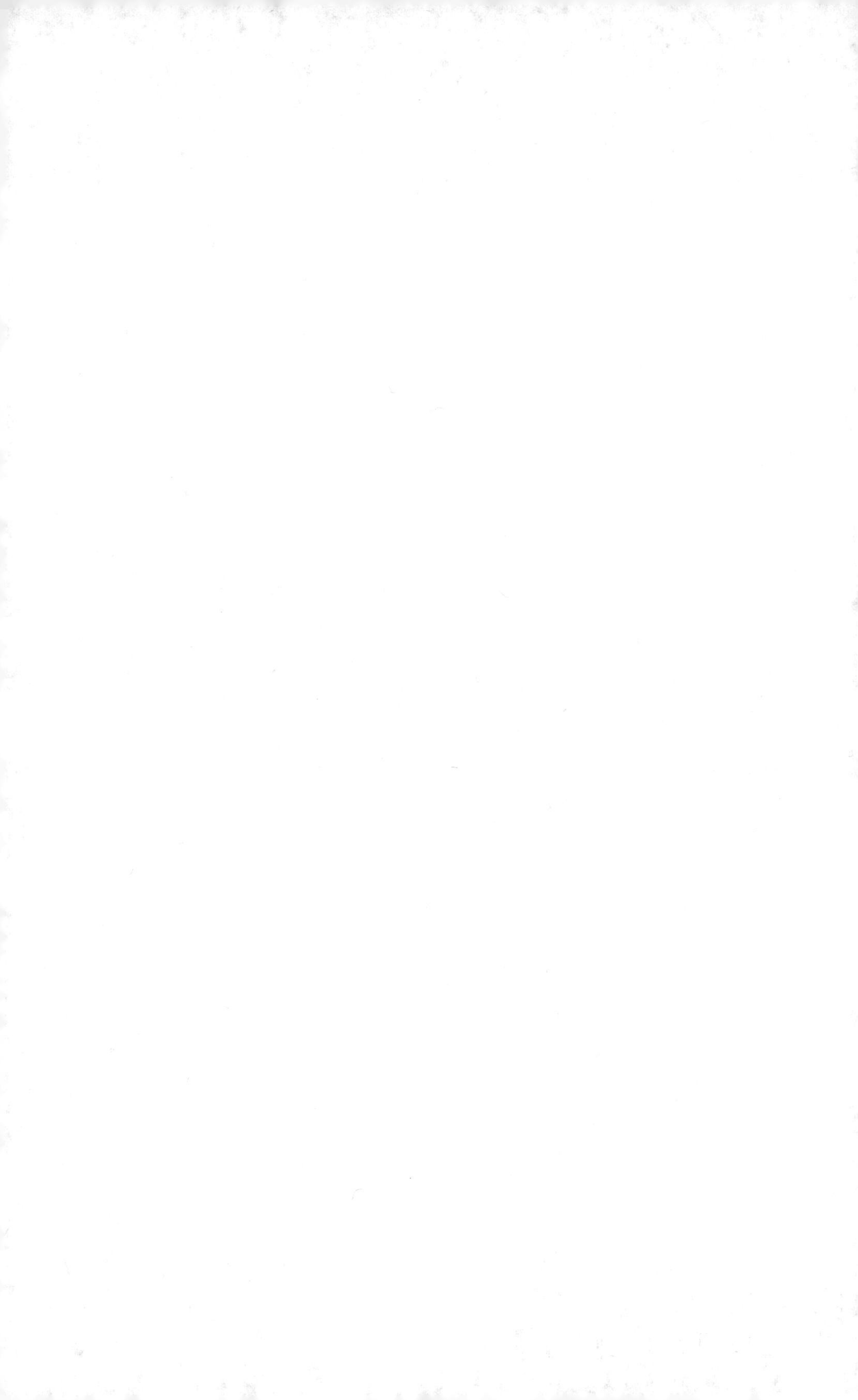

www.ingramcontent.com/pod-product-compliance
Lightning Source LLC
Chambersburg PA
CBHW061619250726
48653CB00034B/2888